Tai-Lormade Books Presents

My Diet, Your Diet

Our Diet

By Nataisha T. Hill

Humble Beginnings

We all know that consumers spend billions of dollars on dieting each year. This includes surgeries, meal programs, diet pills, personal trainers, exercise machines, or anything else that shaves off weight. Sometimes our doctors, peers, lovers, or family members can be first to bring weight gain to our attention before we notice or even care to pay attention to the body changes. Also, who and what we see on television and in magazines sometimes give us the preconceived notion that we're overweight which is why a lot of us resort to desperate measures.

I had a co-worker that wanted to lose weight as quickly as possible, so he ate **only** soup for a week and a half in order to do it. He lost about 12-15 pounds after he was done, but he was delirious and could not function normally at work. He said he would never do that diet again. Then, there is the fact when women have children we rapidly gain weight. Sometimes the career we choose could be a major determination in our size. For instance, sitting at a desk job throughout the day versus someone who is a waitress at a restaurant could make a huge difference in how much weight a person gains over time.

The Charts

Whatever the reason or cause you want to lose weight, there are non-surgical and inexpensive ways to achieve your weight loss goal. I have been well over 200 pounds twice within a few years and I am only about 5 foot 6 inches tall. Chances are if you are my height or shorter and weigh the same 200 pounds or more, then you are probably overweight.

These overweight sizes to height ratios are not composed from my personal standards, but from nutritional weight monitoring charts that I have studied online and in health books. For example, the average woman's height is around 5 foot 4 inches. Therefore, rather you have a small, medium, or large frame; your ideal weight should not exceed around 150 pounds.

First things first, do not panic. According to the same nutritionists, about 70% or more of Americans are overweight. It is also a known fact that the more you age, your metabolism slows down. At about 5 foot 6 inches with a medium frame, my personal goal was to weigh anywhere from 155-165 pounds at maximum weight. Some nutritionists may believe that is still too big for my height, since my ideal weight according to the standard weight chart is set from 130-145 pounds, but this size is what makes me feel sexy and comfortable. Feeling comfortable and attractive at **your** desired weight should be the first step at your weight loss goal. It is okay to be confident and always find ways to compliment other aspects of your appearance even if you are not completely happy with your weight.

For instance, when I was well over weight, considered obese by standards, I definitely made sure my hair, nails, skin, and the little makeup I did wear was on point. Keeping up these physical attributes helped me to maintain what physical confidence I did have about myself and made me want to build on that confidence. In other words, start from the inside out and you may discover losing weight is not something you necessarily want, but just know that being overweight causes more serious health problems such as high blood pressure, which could lead to strokes and heart disease. More importantly, try to have a good support system around to help keep you motivated.

However, try to keep it realistic. Do not say you are comfortable just to cop out and never put forth the effort to even try to lose weight. Many people, especially women, will sometimes say they feel fine and sexy being overweight. Sometimes this perception comes from believing their weight loss goal is not achievable or they have been overweight their entire lives. There are more ways to get 10 than just by adding 5+5. If one diet plan does not work for you or you have been, overweight since you were a child simply means you may have to try different strategies and alternatives to achieve the size you desire.

A Brief History

Most of my life, I was always teased for being too skinny. I hated when people teased me by saying I could fit through door cracks and I looked like a bag of bones. I was about 125 pounds, still around 5 foot 6 inches, and I got up to 132 pounds at the most. I was teased so bad to a point where I started drinking ensure supplemental drinks to help me gain weight. I ate as much as I could, when I could, but nothing helped me gain weight. It was not until well after high school when I embraced my small frame and started modeling. The agency that I joined loved my small frame and the manager's daughter often complimented me about my tiny figure. I did a few amateur gigs, nothing fancy, but modeling definitely helped me to build self-confidence about my body. The beauty of it all was that I could still eat anything I wanted and never gain a pound. Little did I know I would endure both ends of the skinny to overweight spectrum.

The First Round

My body took a toll once I was pregnant with my first child. It was my junior year at a University and even though I was only a few years older than what I thought most students were, I felt embarrassed walking on campus in front of everyone. Obviously, I was having a child but at the same time, I felt fat and the further along I got, the more unattractive I felt. I felt like people were whispering about me being huge and secretly making fun of me while calling me names like beached whale or hippopotamus butt. I know that part of the problem was my insecurity that initially developed overtime from being too skinny. Once I sort of got over that issue, the new problem that then developed was the total opposite, it was a fear of being called, too fat. It only made matters worse when people would ask was I having twins. As mentioned, I was accustomed to being around 125 or 132 pounds at most, so once my weight reached 185 pounds by the end of my second trimester, I decided to register for all online classes that following semester in January since I knew I would only get bigger. More importantly, my baby was also due that February, so I figured it would be the smartest decision. By the time I reached 37 weeks, I was already about 212 pounds. I even skipped my last few appointments at the doctor's office, not only because I did not feel like being weighed, but mainly because my newly added weight kept me exhausted. If I were guessing, I would probably say I was a little over 217 pounds by the time I reached 40 weeks.

After the Pregnancy

I was excited about my baby, but mentally and physically depressed about my weight. I did not want to do any crazy diets like the one I mentioned earlier that my co-worker did since I was breastfeeding and I knew I had to eat healthy for the baby. I wanted to lose weight and I wanted to lose it as quickly as possible. Although about 8 to 10 pounds had come off after the delivery from just the baby's weight alone, I was very unhappy with my 205 or so pound body and everything that came with it. It seemed that everything was physically out of proportion and I did not have the emotional support I felt I needed.

Of course, my mom was my hero who helped tremendously with the baby after my baby was born, but I did not have the type of emotional support where someone would instill in me that I was still beautiful regardless of the weight I gained. I think that feeling alone from a romantic standpoint made me that much more eager or even desperate to lose the weight. To be honest, I was in no hurry to get back on the dating scene, but like anyone else, I wanted to be at my best whenever I did make the decision to start dating.

Trial and Error

I searched dozens of ideas to help me lose weight, but I could only afford so many options since I was a single mom with a newborn. However, I was willing to do whatever it took to get back to what weight I felt was normal. The first method of weight loss I tried was body wraps. I had read that this was not only good for weight loss but aided in the reduction of the appearance of stretch marks as well. I already had most of the ingredients in my cabinet, so expenses were minimal for this weight loss experiment.

For this method, I would sometimes use vapor rub, shea butter, cocoa butter, coconut oil and unbelievably, I even tried peanut butter underneath the wrap. Peanuts contain vitamin E and have properties that aid in cell regeneration. I also used a variety of different homemade scrubs to exfoliate the skin with the wraps as well. Salt, sugar, and essentially anything grainy can be made into a scrub along with most of the listed additives above, however, I would only use the vapor rub alone when adding it underneath my wraps. I sometimes added coffee grinds with the shea butter, which can get very messy. I would apply the ingredient or sometimes a mixture of them together, wrap my entire abdominal section with plastic wrap, and exercise for at least 30-45 minutes with my homemade workout.

The Homemade Workout

My at home workout included anywhere from three to five sets of 20 repetitious exercises. Examples of the exercises I chose were 20 squats, 20 leg lunges, 20 stomach curls, and 20 jumping jacks. I did all exercises in no specific order and finished my exercise routine off by jogging in place. However, some nights the same old routine would bore me, so I would choose about 8-10 different songs that were at least four minutes long and dance until the playlist ended. It was just my baby and I so I could do any dance I wanted without feeling embarrassed. I lived in a one-bedroom townhouse so the staircase was an added bonus before bedtime.

The Real Workout

School started back a few months later and I probably shed another 10 pounds from my homemade workout, so I was still around 193 pounds before stepping foot back onto the university. Along with an entirely different set of new responsibilities, I was still adamant about losing more pounds. On Monday, Wednesday, and Friday I started my mornings off by getting ready, waking my baby and getting her ready, then feeding her before driving her to daycare. I did not have time to eat in the morning, which is something I do not personally recommend, but I did buy chocolate equate breakfast drinks as a substitute. I went to school and once I parked, I had to walk around the entire campus to get to my work-study and the four classes I had throughout the day. Here is the break down for people who may not have an idea of what walking is like on a huge university campus. It took about seven minutes to get to my work-study from the parking lot. The work-study building had a flight of stairs, which I walked every day. There was about a seven-minute increment from my work-study to my first class. The second class was across campus, which was about 12 minutes away and then the 12 minutes from the second class back to a different building where I had my third class on the third floor. I assumed there was an elevator somewhere in that building but I never found it.

The fourth class was a modern dance class, which was technically off campus, so I had to walk back to my car, drive across the main campus area, find another park at the remote building, and walk a little more. I walked roughly about 45 to 50 minutes a day without really noticing. That did not include the warm-ups we had to do in my modern dance class. Besides a hot pocket or lunchable pack here and there, most of the time I didn't get to fully eat until I got home around 4pm, which again, I wouldn't recommend, but my body got used to the routine.

Meal Time

Even though I was eating one full meal a day, I did not have big portions. I would make a box of hamburger helper, meatloaf, or taco salad that would normally be the next day dinner as well, and one side dish. I went out my way to cut back on starches, so my normal side dishes were vegetables that included a choice of sweet peas, green beans, corn, or spinach. I also stayed away from sodas, so juices, milk, and flavored water were solely my drinks. Tuesdays and Thursdays were easier since I only had one class and the work-study, so normally I got a chance to eat a light lunch such as a sandwich and (maybe) a bag of chips here and there to treat myself.

After about 3 or 4 weeks of tiring myself out from school, my work-study, and raising a newborn, I only did my homemade workout on Tuesday and Thursday nights. I would say within a month's time, I had lost about 12 to 15 pounds. Over time, I cut my home workout even shorter, but after the semester ended, which is about a total of 4.5 months, I was back down to 152 pounds.

The Outcome

In a way, I would say this weight loss was definitely the easiest. I was so consumed by having my first child, school, and taking care of everything on my own that I feel that stress played a major role in helping me lose the weight. The miles of walking I was doing throughout the day along with flights of stairs I had to walk up and down definitely took working out to the next level. Again, I would not recommend that you eat practically once a day, but surely cutting back to light meals and at least 30 to 45 minutes of walking or light jogging would help.

This was my first natural diet without weight loss pills, joining a weight-loss program, or any extras, but would not be my last journey to losing weight. What I did to lose weight my first pregnancy would be very different from my second time at dieting. Remember what works for me or someone else may not work for you, so be open to try several different options.

The Second Round

The disappointing thing about losing weight is that it does not stay off by itself. You have to continually work at maintaining your desired weight even when you are finally there. In all honesty, what most people do, including myself, is that we start to get comfortable and fall back into bad habits. You begin to say to yourself that you can have those loaded cheese fries and you stop working out a few days that eventually turns into weeks. Without noticing, you put back on 10 pounds in less than a month. It's human nature and it's exactly what I did the second time around.

The Sitting Job

My first year out of college was a drag and I got a job as a waitress at a popular restaurant. The bad part about working at this particular restaurant was that I loved the food. I would eat before my shift, during lunch, and after my shift. On the contrary, I exercised the calories off whatever I ate running from table to table. At that point, it was a win-win situation. I had chefs cooking delicious foods for me and I was still getting a vigorous exercise for multiple hours, especially when I worked double shifts.

My weight did not undergo another drastic change until I got my office job about a year or so later. I strictly worked sitting down on the phone at my desk. There was absolutely no lifting, pulling, pushing, walking, or any of the sorts required until, of course, I went on break or went home for the day. Furthermore, we had vendors that would bring lunch to the job for employees to purchase and sometimes the company would even buy us lunch. In other words, sitting on the phone all day ultimately made me snack all day as well. We had an indoor workout area in our building that I did not utilize and me working out at home became extinct.

Within about four years of sitting at a desk, I went from a size 7/8 to about a size 14. Yes people, I gained about 40+ pounds. Even though at the time I was still in my late twenties, the weight gain did not bother me because I was comfortable and the people around me that were also around my age were generally the same size or bigger. By this time, I had also gotten married to a husband who loves to cook. Lord knows there is nothing better than having your food prepared for you on almost a daily basis.

My Second Pregnancy

I clearly knew I gained weight by not exercising or being able to fit in my normal clothes, but I honestly was comfortable. It was not until my brother, who I had not seen in a while, made a comment on how big I had gotten. I was accustomed to sibling teasing, but as a married woman, I wondered if my husband secretly felt the same way, though he would not ever tell me. I said to myself it would not hurt if I lost a few pounds and toned up, but as soon as I made a conscience decision to diet again, I got pregnant.

There were positives and one negative about being pregnant for the second time. On a good note, I was married to a great man, my finances were in better order, and my mental and emotional state were better prepared for my second child, but unfortunately, I was physically bigger and in worse shape than ever. I weighed around 150 pounds at the beginning of my first pregnancy, but I weighed in at 190 pounds at the beginning of my second baby. I knew I had to work harder to keep the weight down since I did not have a huge campus to walk and I was not a waitress.

Oddly enough, I was mostly nauseous during my first three months of this pregnancy. I could not hold anything down my stomach to a point where my doctor had to give me medication. Sure enough, the moment passed and I was back on a highway to heavy. My mind would say 'go walking in the park' but my body said 'rest, grab a snack, and watch a good show'. Ultimately, after listening to my body over the last two trimesters, my last weigh in before the delivery was 252 pounds.

After the Second Pregnancy

Unlike my first pregnancy, the emotional support after I had the baby was great. I was on maternity leave from work for six weeks, so I figured I had to at least lose 15 to 20 pounds before going back to work. My baby was 9 pounds and 4 ounces, so about 10 pounds came off immediately after delivery. Although I did not see it, my husband would tell me I was beautiful regardless of the weight. In my mind, I felt as if he felt complimenting me was something he was required to do. While I appreciated his compliments, I felt unattractive to myself. I wanted to not only feel sexy, but also look sexy in the mirror.

I took the time for my body to heal and get my newborn on a routine before returning to work. Although I lost an additional 10 pounds from not having a good appetite for about 3-4 weeks, I still could not fit in any of my favorite jeans, which were my favorite article of clothing. Besides the fact that the majority of my jeans were around a size of 9/10, most of the sizes in the brands and styles that I wore only went up to about size 12 to my knowledge. Perhaps this theory only applied to the particular stores of where I shopped, but I felt at a lost. Determined not to buy an entire new wardrobe, change up my style, or where I shopped, I had no other option but to lose the weight.

As I returned to work, my appetite also returned and I was probably eating two full meals a day, lunch and dinner, and I would snack in between. I still did not normally eat breakfast. My idea of a full meal at the time was a meat (could be two meats if it was chicken or fish) two sides, a drink (normally soda) and a dessert. My ideal snacks were chips, cakes, cookies, and other unhealthy foods. I felt myself falling back into the same routine that made me gain weight before the pregnancy and trust me; nothing is more insulting than someone to ask you 'when are you due' when you are no longer pregnant.

Getting the Weight Off

My first attempt to take the weight off was by joining a weight loss center. I think I paid 90 dollars for the consultation and the nurse gave me a brief physical exam to help determine my weight loss goal. They also gave me written dieting suggestions and a 30-day prescription of weight loss pills. I was assuming like any diet pill, it would help to suppress my appetite and help rebuild my energy. Unfortunately, taking the diet pill gave me a headache along with jitters, uncontrollable movement in my hands. I discarded the bottle after trying the pills for about three consecutive days.

Still determined to get the weight off, I researched natural approaches to dieting. This is when I discovered the beauty of a waist-trainer. The first one I ordered online was a size too small. The idea in my mind was to order a size down to make it fit tighter. This was and still is a terrible idea. Most good waist-trainers have three adjustable sizes designed to fit your waist as you lose weight. Take it from me; order your correct size even if you feel some type of way from having to order a size 3x or larger.

Once I received my second waist-trainer, I immediately attempted to secure it around my abdominal section. I literally had to lie down on my back in order to fasten all the metal loops. The waist-trainer definitely squeezed my entire abdominal area together and I was able to breathe naturally. This bit of extra information sounds silly, but is very important. I have read in articles that some people have blacked out or fainted from wearing a waist-trainer that obstructed their breathing, so be mindful of your lungs. I kept the trainer on for about an hour after doing a little housework. Although it was a relief to take it off, I felt like I had accomplished something since the entire area that was consumed inside the trainer was wet from sweat.

I continued to do one hour of waist training while I was at home for about a week. I bumped it up to about 3 hours the next week and added pushing my baby in the stroller around the neighborhood to my routine. I did not know how I would feel wearing it to work, so I still only wore the trainer at home. I noticed it was a lot easier to put on around the end of the third week, so I assumed it had stretch to accommodate my size. I did not get on the scale to check to see if I had lost weight because I did not want to be disappointed had I not lost any pounds.

A little after a month of consistently wearing the trainer, I finally started wearing it to work 2 or 3 times a week for 8 hours a day. I have to admit it was a little uncomfortable in the beginning and I think I only wore it half a day the first time, but I loved the way I appeared much slimmer as if I had an hourglass shape.

I decided to give myself a break close to the two-month mark and just put on regular clothes without the trainer underneath. Low and behold, I did not have to struggle to fit into the few pair of jeans I was able to wear at the time. This small victory prompted me to check the scale and I discovered I had lost about 10 pounds. This further inspired me to keep pushing.

Bumping up the Routine

A group of co-workers and I decided to join a fitness center at a discounted rate. The center took off $10 per monthly admission if eight of us joined. The ambience of the center was very nice. There was a lap pool outside, a steam room, an upstairs track, basketball court, tennis room, and daily workout classes such as Zumba, Hip-hop dance, and yoga that were free with the membership. I took a few dance classes, walked the track, and did one muscle-building session.

After my first month, my time seemed more limited and I stopped dedicating myself to go. I probably did a week worth of visits altogether and basically gave the fitness center a free $160 for holding a membership "just in case" I decided to return at some point. Unfortunately, I never returned and terminated the membership several months later.

My Ultimate Salvation

By popular demand, I decided to add apple cider vinegar to my daily regimen. Apple cider vinegar helps clean out bacteria in your system, suppress your appetite, and speeds up your metabolism by increasing your energy. Apple cider vinegar is also an excellent detoxifying agent for your body.

I knew the smell of apple cider vinegar was repulsive, so the taste could not be too much different. Common sense and as instructed, told me to dilute whatever intake I could stomach. I took a medicine-measuring cup, poured in 2ml of apple cider vinegar, added a tsp of honey, about 5 drops of lemon juice, and about 2 ounces of water. I chose a small amount to see how my body would react to it and I tried this experiment on a morning of my day off just in case it caused adverse reactions. Much to my surprise, I did not get an upset stomach, but I did have an urgent bowel movement a few hours later. I read an article that stated to add cinnamon to the blend to help extract the overwhelming taste and for cinnamon's known antioxidants, but I normally would not remember until after I had already chugged down the initial mixture.

I made a commitment to do this same routine every morning regardless of the taste. Sometimes I would hold my nose to drown out the taste even after I added the honey. After about 2 and a half or 3 weeks, I increase my intake from 2ml to 4ml. I did not increase the honey or lemon intake, but I did add a chaser, which was a shot glass of Apple juice after I drank the mixture. The fact of the matter was even though my daily intake was consistent; I never got use to the taste.

Meal Time

As I mentioned earlier, I have never been an adamant breakfast eater. I still ate lunch and dinner, but there were noticeable changes in my appetite by adding apple cider vinegar to my diet. When I would eat my lunch, I could not finish the entire meal as I once did. I would literally end up discarding almost half of my meal. This applied to both lunch and dinner, so I started buying and eating smaller portions. Believe it or not, a kid's meal would feel my stomach!

I also would still eat regular foods and soul food such as lasagna, chicken and dressing, spaghetti, wings, cheeseburgers, roast beef, and all kinds of other delicious foods. The key for me was eating the smaller portions of whatever I chose to eat. I think around this time, which was about 2 months after I starting drinking the vinegar, I lost around another 12 to 15 pounds. I also stopped wearing the waist trainer and only brought it out on formal wear occasions.

Upping the Antics Once Again

In addition to the vinegar, I added the fit-bit wristband to my daily routine as well. A good friend of mine was also trying to lose weight, so she told me about a group of women who compete for most steps. I was interested at the least, but I did want to support her on her weight lost journey. Much to my surprise, I became addicted to the challenges. There is an automatic moderator on an app that you download onto your phone that lets you know when you are in the lead, when someone is catching up, or when you reach a milestone. It allows you to encourage others and send messages to those in your group. The app also monitors your calories by inputting your foods, your sleep, your heart rate, tracks your steps, and so much more. The information you enter regarding your weight loss goal is private so no one in the group can see your personal stats.

It was something about the gratification of being announced number one to other group members although it was all in good fun to lose weight. I would find myself getting up in the middle of the night just to keep my lead. I am not a spokesperson for fit-bit, but this definitely became an enjoyable way for me to get healthy and I recommend it for any group of friends who would like to lose weight together.

The Results

As unfortunate this may be to readers, I honestly did not keep an exact timeline of my weight loss progression once my baby started being mobile everywhere in the home. I would "guesstimate" and say I lost an additional 20 pounds in the course of 2-3 months using a combination of the vinegar and fit-bit challenges. I can say that by the time I got down from 200 pounds to around 178 pounds, I continued to lose weight at a gradual pace. So again, if I go out on a limb, I would say I lost about 50-60 pounds over 9 to 11 months without any vigorous exercising.

My Advice

I would say my key to success at losing weight came from trying different options. I was not afraid to try something new and I was not afraid to let something go if I felt it did not work for me. I feel another important lesson is not to give up. I know we like instant gratification when it comes to getting down to a desired size, but obviously the same time it took to gain it, will likely be the equivalent time it will take to lose it unless you indulge in the idea of surgery. I honestly could have gotten quicker results had I dedicated myself to a consistent workout routine everyday and ate healthier foods such as salmon, tuna, chicken breast, fruits and vegetables, or foods low in sodium and sugar in addition to my diets, but I did not. Overall, once you do find that special something that works for you, stay consistent, try to keep encouraging people in your circle, and stay positive.

Good Luck and Best of Wishes

www.ingramcontent.com/pod-product-compliance
Lightning Source LLC
Chambersburg PA
CBHW021344290326
41933CB00037B/725